THE MENOPAUSE RENEWAL

Eliminate Your Symptoms and Rediscover Your Younger Self Once More

By

Dr. Nina Lowe

contents of this book and specifically disclaim any implied warranties of merchantability or fitness for a particular purpose. The author and publisher shall not be held liable for any loss or damages whatsoever arising from, or in connection with, the use of this book.

This book is intended for informational purposes only. The author and publisher do not offer any medical, legal, or professional advice. If you require such advice, please seek the services of a competent professional.

Table of contents

Introduction

The journey through menopause is a profound transitional phase that every woman encounters—a natural progression signaling the end of one chapter and the beginning of another. This pivotal time brings with it a symphony of changes, both internal and external, that can be as complex as they are transformative. "The Menopause Renewal" is your compass for navigating this journey, providing a roadmap to not only navigate challenges but also embrace newfound opportunities for growth, wisdom, and empowerment.

Menopause is a multifaceted experience, encompassing a wide spectrum of physical, emotional, and psychological shifts. It's a period where the body's hormonal landscape undergoes a metamorphosis, triggering a cascade of changes that reverberate through every facet of life. The cessation of menstruation marks an end to one's reproductive years, and while this may signal a sense of loss for some, it's essential to remember that it also heralds the dawn of a new era—one characterized by self-discovery, resilience, and renewed purpose.

"The Menopause Renewal" is your guide to understanding the science underpinning these transformations. Through the lens of biology and physiology, we'll uncover the intricate interplay of hormones, demystifying the processes that govern your body. From the fluctuations in estrogen levels to the impact on bone health and metabolism, we'll unravel the complexities that define this phase. This knowledge empowers you to approach menopause armed with a deeper understanding of your body's needs, laying the foundation for informed decisions about your well-being.

One of the hallmarks of menopause is the diverse array of symptoms that may arise, ranging from the infamous hot flashes and night sweats to mood swings, sleep disturbances, and changes in cognitive function. "The Menopause Renewal" provides practical strategies to navigate these challenges. We delve into evidence-based approaches to manage and mitigate symptoms, allowing you to regain control over your life and well-being. By offering insights into hormone therapy and alternative remedies, we enable you to make choices that align with your unique journey.

However, menopause extends beyond the physiological realm. It's an opportunity to delve into your emotional landscape, fostering a deeper connection with yourself. As you traverse the terrains of mood swings, anxiety, and self-discovery, this guide offers strategies to nurture emotional well-being. By embracing self-care practices, enhancing your emotional resilience, and nurturing healthy relationships, you can cultivate an empowered mindset that accompanies you throughout this transformative passage.

Nutrition and fitness play pivotal roles in sculpting your menopausal experience. "The Menopause Renewal" offers a comprehensive exploration of how diet and exercise can support hormonal balance and overall well-being. From nourishing your body with hormone-supportive foods to crafting exercise routines that bolster bone health, cardiovascular fitness, and mental clarity, this guide empowers you to embrace a holistic approach to wellness.

"The Menopause Renewal" recognizes that this phase is a unique canvas upon which you can paint a vivid tapestry of beauty and confidence. With practical advice on skincare, fashion, and embracing self-love, we guide you in embracing the changes that come with age. It's a celebration of the wisdom that accompanies each passing year, a testament to the vibrant spirit that continues to evolve and thrive.

In this book, you'll find not just insights, but a transformative journey that transcends the confines of biology. "The Menopause Renewal" is an invitation to reconnect with your body, rekindle your passions, and embrace your authentic self. As you traverse the pages ahead, remember that this guide is your companion—an unwavering presence to lean on during moments of uncertainty, a source of inspiration during times of change, and a beacon of empowerment guiding you toward a revitalized sense of well-being.

Menopause is not an ending; it's a bridge to a new beginning. It's an opportunity to redefine your relationship with yourself, uncover latent strengths, and bask in the radiance of your uniqueness. With "The Menopause Renewal," embark on this transformative journey armed with knowledge, compassion, and the tools to craft a menopause experience that is uniquely yours.

Chapter 1

The Science of Menopause

Menopause, a universal biological phenomenon experienced by women, marks a significant transition in a woman's life journey. It is not merely an endpoint but a complex process governed by intricate hormonal and physiological changes. Understanding the science behind menopause is crucial not only for comprehending the physical shifts that occur but also for navigating this period with grace and empowerment.

Hormonal Orchestra

At the heart of menopause lies a symphony of hormonal changes that cascade through a woman's body. The ovaries, which have been the primary source of estrogen and progesterone, start to produce these hormones in dwindling amounts as menopause approaches. Estrogen, a key player in the menstrual cycle, exerts its influence on various body systems, including the reproductive, cardiovascular, and skeletal systems.

As estrogen levels decrease, a series of events unfold. Menstrual cycles become irregular, eventually ceasing altogether. Follicle-stimulating hormone (FSH) and luteinizing hormone (LH), both produced by the pituitary gland, surge in response to lower estrogen levels. These hormonal shifts underpin the physiological changes that define menopause.

Perimenopause

Before the final cessation of menstruation, women undergo a transitional phase known as perimenopause. This period, often marked by irregular periods and varying hormone levels, can last for several years. It's during perimenopause that many of the well-known symptoms of menopause, such as hot flashes and mood swings, make their debut.

During perimenopause, the ovaries continue to produce estrogen, but in an erratic manner. This unpredictability contributes to hormonal fluctuations that can trigger an array of symptoms. While these changes might seem disruptive, they are a natural reflection of the body's adaptation to its changing hormonal landscape.

<u>Hot Flashes and Hormonal Havoc</u>

Hot flashes are one of the most recognizable and frequently reported symptoms of menopause. These sudden, intense waves of heat can cause flushing, sweating, and discomfort. They are believed to be triggered by changes in the hypothalamus, a region of the brain that regulates body temperature. Fluctuating hormone levels, particularly estrogen, are thought to play a role in disrupting the hypothalamus's temperature control mechanisms.

However, hot flashes are not solely attributed to estrogen. Neurotransmitters such as norepinephrine and serotonin also influence the frequency and intensity of hot flashes. The intricate interplay between hormones and neural signaling contributes to the variability in hot flashes experiences among women.

Mood Swings and Emotional Rollercoasters

Hormonal shifts during menopause can have a significant impact on mood and emotional well-being. Fluctuations in estrogen levels have been linked to mood swings, irritability, and even increased vulnerability to anxiety and depression. Understanding these emotional changes is essential, as it helps women recognize the connection between their mental health and hormonal fluctuations. By embracing self-care practices, seeking support, and considering various therapeutic approaches, women can navigate the emotional challenges of menopause with resilience and grace.

Metabolism in Flux

The hormonal changes that occur during menopause can influence metabolism and body composition. As estrogen levels decline, some women may experience weight gain, particularly around the abdominal area. This shift can be attributed to changes in how the body stores and uses energy. Combating weight gain during menopause requires a multifaceted approach that includes a balanced diet, regular exercise, and an awareness of the body's changing nutritional needs.

Cognitive Changes

Cognitive changes during menopause often lead to concerns about memory and concentration. While the exact relationship between estrogen and cognitive function is still being studied, it's clear that hormonal fluctuations can influence brain activity. Estrogen receptors are present in brain regions responsible for memory and mood regulation, indicating a potential connection between hormonal shifts and cognitive changes.

The "menopausal fog" experienced by some women could be attributed to these hormonal fluctuations, but it's important to note that cognitive changes are highly individual. Factors such as sleep quality, stress levels, and overall health also contribute to cognitive function during this period.

<u>Bone Health</u>

Beyond its impact on reproductive function, estrogen plays a crucial role in maintaining bone density. As estrogen levels decline, the risk of osteoporosis—a condition characterized by weakened bones—increases. This heightened risk underscores the importance of maintaining bone health through lifestyle modifications and, in some cases, medical interventions.

Exercise, particularly weight-bearing and resistance training, can help mitigate bone loss and maintain bone strength. Calcium and vitamin D intake also play a pivotal role in supporting bone health. The understanding of the hormonal and physiological mechanisms involved in bone health during menopause underscores the significance of a holistic approach to well-being.

Cardiovascular Health

Menopause is also associated with shifts in cardiovascular health. Estrogen has a protective effect on the cardiovascular system, promoting healthy blood vessel function and lipid profiles. As estrogen levels decrease, these protective effects diminish, increasing the risk of cardiovascular diseases.

Understanding these cardiovascular changes is crucial for proactive health management. Lifestyle adjustments, including a heart-healthy diet, regular exercise, and stress reduction techniques, can mitigate some of the cardiovascular risks associated with menopause.

The science of menopause reveals the intricacies of a woman's body as it undergoes a remarkable transformation. Hormonal fluctuations, including the decline of estrogen, influence a range of physiological systems and give rise to a diverse array of symptoms. From hot flashes to cognitive changes and cardiovascular shifts, menopause is a holistic experience that demands a comprehensive approach to well-being.

Navigating menopause armed with knowledge empowers women to make informed decisions about their health and lifestyle. It's important to recognize that menopause is not a one-size-fits-all experience; each woman's journey is unique. By understanding the science underpinning these changes, women can embrace the menopause as a transformative passage—one that offers the opportunity for growth, self-discovery, and empowerment.

Chapter 2

Navigating Symptoms

Menopause, often referred to as a "change of life," signifies the conclusion of a woman's reproductive journey. This natural transition is accompanied by a myriad of physical, emotional, and psychological changes. The symphony of symptoms that arises during menopause is a testament to the intricate interplay of hormones, genetics, lifestyle, and individual experiences. Navigating these symptoms is a transformative journey that requires a holistic understanding and a tailored approach.

Hot Flashes and Night Sweats

Hot flashes and night sweats are two of the most characteristic and widely recognized symptoms of menopause. Hot flashes are characterized by a sudden sensation of heat spreading throughout the body, often accompanied by flushed skin and sweating. Night sweats are essentially hot flashes that occur during sleep, leading to disrupted sleep patterns.

The exact cause of hot flashes and night sweats is still not fully understood, but hormonal fluctuations, particularly the decline in estrogen levels, are believed to play a central role. The hypothalamus, a region of the brain responsible for regulating body temperature, seems to be sensitive to these hormonal shifts. When estrogen levels fluctuate, the hypothalamus may mistakenly perceive the body as overheating, triggering the body's cooling mechanisms.

Managing hot flashes and night sweats involves a combination of lifestyle adjustments and behavioral strategies:

1. Dress in Layers: Wearing lightweight and breathable clothing in layers allows you to easily adapt to temperature changes.

2. Stay Hydrated: Drinking plenty of water helps regulate body temperature and mitigate the intensity of hot flashes.

3. Mindful Breathing and Relaxation Techniques: Deep breathing exercises and relaxation practices can help reduce the frequency and intensity of hot flashes.

4. Cooling Measures: Keeping a fan nearby, using cooling pillows, and maintaining a cooler sleeping environment can alleviate night sweats.

Mood Swings and Emotional Well-Being

Mood swings, irritability, anxiety, and even depression are common emotional experiences during menopause. Hormonal fluctuations certainly contribute to these mood changes, but they are not the sole factor. Other elements, such as sleep disturbances, lifestyle adjustments, and psychological responses to the transition, also play a role.

Managing emotional well-being during menopause involves addressing both physiological and psychological aspects:

1. Mindfulness and Meditation: Practices that promote mindfulness and meditation can help manage stress and anxiety.

2. Supportive Social Connections: Engaging with friends, family, or support groups provides emotional outlets.

3. Professional Help: For persistent mood disturbances, seeking therapy or counseling can offer valuable support.

Sleep Disruptions

Sleep disturbances are a common complaint during menopause. Women often experience difficulties falling asleep, staying asleep, or experiencing restful sleep. Hormonal fluctuations, night sweats, and changes in sleep architecture contribute to these disruptions.

Improving sleep quality during menopause involves adopting sleep-friendly habits:

1. Create a Sleep Schedule: Maintaining consistent bedtime and wake-up times assists in regulating the body's internal rhythm.

2. Create a Sleep-Conducive Environment: Dark, cool, and quiet bedrooms promote better sleep.

3. Reduce Screen Usage Before Sleep: Engaging with screens before bedtime can disturb sleep cycles.

4. Avoid Heavy Meals and Caffeine Close to Bedtime: These can interfere with sleep.

<u>Weight Management</u>

Weight management becomes a more complex endeavor during menopause. Metabolism tends to slow down, and hormonal changes can lead to an increase in fat accumulation, particularly around the abdomen.

Approaches to maintaining a healthy weight during menopause include:

1. Balanced Diet: Prioritize nutrient-dense foods and practice portion control.

2. Regular Exercise: Participate in a combination of cardiovascular workouts, strength training, and flexibility exercises.

3. Stress Management: Chronic stress can contribute to weight gain, so adopting stress-reduction techniques is important.

Cognitive Changes

Cognitive changes, such as memory lapses and difficulty concentrating, are often reported during menopause.

While the relationship between hormonal changes and cognitive function is not yet fully understood, several factors contribute to these changes.

Supporting cognitive function involves a multifaceted approach:

1. Brain-Boosting Activities: Engage in puzzles, and games, and learn new skills to stimulate the brain.

2. Healthy Lifestyle: Regular exercise, a balanced diet, and quality sleep all support cognitive health.

3. Mental Health Care: Addressing stress, anxiety, and mood disturbances can positively impact cognitive function.

The journey through menopause is a transformative experience that demands a comprehensive approach to well-being. Navigating symptoms requires an understanding of the complex interplay between hormones, lifestyle, and individual responses. By embracing the changes as a natural aspect of the life cycle and applying strategies to manage symptoms, women can navigate menopause with grace, resilience, and empowerment.

Each woman's menopausal journey is unique, and it's important to approach it with self-compassion and flexibility. The symptoms that arise during this time are not an indication of weakness; rather, they are a testament to the body's remarkable adaptability. By fostering physical well-being through lifestyle adjustments, nurturing emotional health, and seeking support when needed, women can navigate the complexities of menopause with a sense of empowerment and confidence.

Remember that menopause is not the end of a chapter but the beginning of a new one—one that offers the opportunity for self-discovery, growth, and renewal. As you navigate the ups and downs of menopause, may you find strength in your journey and embrace this period of transformation with an open heart and a resilient spirit.

Chapter 3

Nutrition for Menopause

Menopause marks a significant transition in a woman's life—one that brings about a cascade of hormonal changes that can impact various aspects of well-being. While this phase is a natural part of the aging process, adopting a balanced and supportive approach to nutrition can play a crucial role in managing symptoms and promoting overall health. Understanding the role of nutrition during menopause and making informed dietary choices empowers women to navigate this transformative journey with vitality and resilience.

The Hormonal Landscape

As women enter menopause, hormonal changes take center stage. One of the primary hormones affected is estrogen, which plays a vital role in bone health, heart health, and metabolism. The decline in estrogen levels during menopause can lead to changes in body composition, bone density reduction, and an increased risk of heart disease.

Maintaining a healthy and balanced diet becomes essential during this phase to provide the body with the necessary nutrients for optimal functioning. Nutrient-rich foods help support bone health, cardiovascular health, and overall well-being.

Essential Nutrients for Menopause

1. Calcium: Adequate calcium intake is crucial for maintaining bone density and preventing osteoporosis. Calcium can be obtained from sources like dairy items, fortified plant-based milks, leafy greens, and almonds, which are all valuable options.

2. Vitamin D: Vitamin D aids in calcium absorption and is essential for bone health. Exposure to sunlight, fortified foods, fatty fish, and supplements can help meet vitamin D needs.

3. Magnesium: This mineral supports bone health, muscle function, and sleep quality. Magnesium can be found abundantly in nuts, seeds, whole grains, and leafy greens, making them excellent sources of this essential mineral.

4. Omega-3 Fatty Acids: Omega-3s have anti-inflammatory properties that can help alleviate symptoms such as joint pain and mood disturbances. Fatty fish (like salmon and mackerel), flaxseeds, and walnuts are rich in omega-3s.

5. Fiber: Fiber aids digestion, supports heart health and helps manage weight. Dietary fiber can be derived from whole grains, legumes, fruits, and vegetables, all of which are outstanding sources of this important nutrient.

6. Phytoestrogens: These plant compounds have a mild estrogenic effect, which can help alleviate certain menopausal symptoms. Phytoestrogens are present in soy products, flaxseeds, and legumes.

<u>Building a Balanced Plate</u>

1. Fruits and Vegetables: A diet rich in colorful fruits and vegetables provide essential vitamins, minerals, and antioxidants. Aim to fill half your plate with these nutrient-packed foods to support overall health.

2. Lean Proteins: Incorporate lean protein sources such as poultry, fish, lean meats, eggs, legumes, and tofu. Protein supports muscle maintenance, immune function, and hormone production.

3. Whole Grains: Opt for whole grains like quinoa, brown rice, oats, and whole wheat bread. These provide sustained energy, fiber, and essential nutrients.

4. Healthy Fats: Incorporate sources of beneficial fats like avocados, nuts, seeds, and olive oil into your diet. These fats promote cardiovascular well-being and contribute to a feeling of fullness.

5. Dairy or Dairy Alternatives: Choose low-fat or fortified dairy products or plant-based alternatives to support calcium and vitamin D intake.

6. Hydration: Maintaining proper hydration is crucial for one's overall state of health. Aim for at least 8 glasses of water a day and consider herbal teas for added variety.

Nutritional Strategies for Menopausal Symptoms

1. Managing Hot Flashes: Some women find that spicy foods and caffeine can trigger hot flashes. Opt for cooling foods like cucumbers, watermelon, and mint to help manage body temperature.

2. Mood Management: Foods rich in B vitamins, such as whole grains, leafy greens, and lean proteins, support mood and energy regulation.

3. Bone Health: Focus on calcium-rich foods and vitamin D sources to support bone density and reduce the risk of osteoporosis.

4. Heart Health: Choose heart-healthy fats, like those found in fatty fish and olive oil, to support cardiovascular well-being.

5. Weight Management: Emphasize whole foods, lean proteins, and fiber-rich options to support weight management during menopause.

6. Gut Health: A diet rich in fiber from fruits, vegetables, and whole grains supports gut health and digestive regularity.

Hormone-Supportive Superfoods

1. Flaxseeds: These are rich in omega-3 fatty acids and lignans, which have potential hormone-balancing effects.

2. Soy: Soy products like tofu and tempeh contain phytoestrogens that may help alleviate certain menopausal symptoms.

3. Cruciferous Vegetables: Broccoli, cauliflower, and Brussels sprouts contain compounds that support hormone metabolism and balance.

4. Berries: Berries are packed with antioxidants that support overall health and aging.

5. Fatty Fish: Fatty fish like salmon provide omega-3s, which have anti-inflammatory benefits and support heart health.

Lifestyle Factors and Mindful Eating

While nutrition is a cornerstone of menopausal health, it's important to complement a balanced diet with mindful eating practices and other lifestyle adjustments:

1. Portion Control: Pay attention to portion sizes to prevent overeating and support weight management.

2. Mindful Eating: Engage in mindful eating by relishing every mouthful, consuming your food at a leisurely pace, and being attuned to signals of both hunger and satisfaction.

3. Regular Physical Activity: Regular exercise supports metabolism, bone health, and overall well-being.

4. Stress Management: Chronic stress can exacerbate menopausal symptoms. Participate in relaxation practices such as meditation, yoga, or practicing deep breathing exercises.

5. Adequate Sleep: Prioritize quality sleep, as it supports hormonal balance and overall health.

Navigating menopause with grace and vitality involves embracing nutrition as a powerful tool for managing symptoms and promoting overall health. By understanding the specific nutrient needs during this phase and making informed dietary choices, women can support bone health, cardiovascular well-being, weight management, and emotional balance. A diet rich in essential nutrients, phytoestrogens, and hormone-supportive superfoods provides a foundation for resilience and empowerment through this transformative journey. Remember, menopause is not a time of limitation but an opportunity to nourish the body and cultivate well-being in new and meaningful ways.

Chapter 4

Fitness and Movement

Menopause ushers in a period of change and transition, both on a physiological and emotional level. Engaging in regular physical activity and adopting a fitness routine tailored to your body's changing needs can have a profound impact on your overall well-being during this transformative phase. Embracing fitness and movement not only helps manage menopausal symptoms but also empowers you to navigate this journey with strength, vitality, and a renewed sense of self.

Understanding the Benefits of Exercise During Menopause

As estrogen levels decline during menopause, various physical changes may occur, including a decrease in bone density, muscle mass, and metabolic rate. However, engaging in regular exercise can counteract these changes and offer numerous benefits:

1. Bone Health: Weight-bearing exercises, such as walking, jogging, and resistance training, help maintain bone density and reduce the risk of osteoporosis.

2. Muscle Maintenance: Strength training exercises preserve muscle mass and help prevent muscle loss that often accompanies aging.

3. Metabolic Boost: Regular exercise supports metabolism and helps manage weight gain, which is common during menopause.

4. Cardiovascular Health: Aerobic exercises, such as swimming, cycling, and dancing, improve cardiovascular fitness and reduce the risk of heart disease.

5. Mood Enhancement: Exercise triggers the release of endorphins, which can alleviate mood swings, anxiety, and depression commonly experienced during menopause.

6. Cognitive Benefits: Physical activity supports cognitive function and may help manage memory changes often associated with menopause.

Designing a Menopause-Friendly Exercise Routine

Creating a fitness routine that suits your individual needs and preferences is essential. It's important to consider your fitness level, any existing health conditions, and your personal goals. Always consult with a healthcare professional before starting a new exercise program, especially if you have any medical concerns.

1. Cardiovascular Exercises

Walking: A low-impact option that can be done anywhere, walking supports cardiovascular health and bone density.

Swimming: Gentle on the joints, swimming provides an effective full-body workout.

Cycling: Whether outdoors or on a stationary bike, cycling improves cardiovascular fitness and lower body strength.

Dancing: Not only is dancing fun, but it also enhances cardiovascular fitness and coordination.

2. Strength Training

Bodyweight Exercises: Push-ups, squats, lunges, and planks are effective bodyweight exercises that build strength.

Resistance Bands: These versatile tools offer gentle resistance to help maintain muscle mass and bone density.

Free Weights: Incorporate dumbbells or kettlebells to perform exercises targeting various muscle groups.

3. Flexibility and Balance

Yoga: Enhances flexibility, balance, and relaxation. Yoga also promotes mindfulness, reducing stress and anxiety.

Pilates: Focuses on core strength, flexibility, and alignment, which are essential for maintaining posture and balance.

4. Interval Training

High-Intensity Interval Training (HIIT): Alternates between intense bursts of activity and short recovery periods, promoting cardiovascular fitness and metabolism.

5. Mind-Body Practices

Tai Chi: This ancient practice combines movement, breath, and meditation to improve balance, flexibility, and mental clarity.

Meditation: Mindfulness meditation can reduce stress, enhance emotional well-being, and promote relaxation.

6. Listening to Your Body

Observe how your body reacts to physical activity. If something causes discomfort or pain, adjust or modify the exercise accordingly.

Give importance to taking days off for rest to enable your body to recuperate and avoid excessive training.

Staying Active Throughout the Day

Incorporating movement into your daily routine goes beyond structured workouts. Simple lifestyle adjustments can help you stay active and energized throughout the day:

1.   Take the Stairs: Opt for stairs instead of elevators to increase daily physical activity.

2. Stretch Breaks: Set a timer to remind yourself to stand up, stretch, and move around every hour.

3. Walk More: Park farther away from your destination or take short walking breaks during your workday.

4. Gardening: Engaging in gardening activities can provide low-impact exercise and connect you with nature.

5. Household Chores: Vacuuming, sweeping, and other household chores contribute to daily movement.

Overcoming Challenges and Staying Motivated

While the benefits of exercise during menopause are vast, challenges can arise. This is how you can maintain your motivation and conquer challenges:

1. Hormonal Fluctuations

Recognize that energy levels may vary during different phases of your menstrual cycle or menopause. Adapt your workouts accordingly.

Prioritize consistency over intensity. Consistent, moderate exercise can be more sustainable than sporadic intense workouts.

2. Joint Health

Choose low-impact activities, such as swimming or cycling, to protect joints while staying active.

Incorporate flexibility exercises to maintain joint mobility and prevent stiffness.

3. Time Constraints

Break exercise into shorter sessions throughout the day. Ten-minute bursts of activity can add up to significant benefits.

Choose activities you enjoy, as you're more likely to make time for them.

4. Emotional Well-Being

Use exercise as a tool to manage stress and improve mood. Engaging in physical activity releases endorphins, which can boost your spirits.

Exercise outdoors whenever possible. Nature and fresh air can have a positive impact on emotional well-being.

Staying Hydrated and Nourished

Consume water prior to, during, and after your workout to ensure proper hydration.

Consume a balanced meal or snack containing carbohydrates and protein after a workout to aid recovery.

Embracing fitness and movement during menopause is a powerful way to enhance your physical, mental, and emotional well-being. Regular physical activity supports bone health, cardiovascular fitness, muscle strength, and overall vitality. Whether it's through cardiovascular exercises, strength training, flexibility practices, or mind-body activities, finding an exercise routine that suits your preferences and needs empowers you to navigate menopause with strength, grace, and resilience.

Remember that your fitness journey is unique, and it's important to listen to your body and make adjustments as needed. Embrace the journey with patience and self-compassion, and celebrate the progress you make along the way. As you engage in fitness and movement, you're not just promoting physical health; you're also nurturing a deeper connection with your body and embracing the incredible journey of menopause with empowerment and confidence.

Chapter 5

Hormone Therapy and Alternatives

Menopause is a significant life transition that brings about a series of hormonal changes. For many women, these changes are accompanied by a range of symptoms that can impact their quality of life. Hormone therapy (HT), also known as hormone replacement therapy (HRT), has long been a standard approach to managing menopausal symptoms. However, there are also alternative options available. Understanding the benefits, risks, and alternatives to hormone therapy empowers women to make informed decisions that align with their individual needs and preferences.

Hormone Therapy

Hormone therapy involves the use of medications containing hormones like estrogen, progesterone, or both, to replace the declining levels of these hormones during menopause. It aims to alleviate menopausal symptoms such as hot flashes, night sweats, vaginal dryness, and mood changes.

Hormone therapy comes in various forms, including pills, patches, creams, gels, and vaginal preparations.

Benefits of Hormone Therapy

1. **Symptom Relief:** Hormone therapy is effective in reducing the frequency and severity of menopausal symptoms, improving the quality of life for many women.

2. **Bone Health:** Estrogen replacement can help prevent bone loss and reduce the risk of osteoporosis.

3. Cardiovascular Protection: For some women, hormone therapy may have a protective effect on the cardiovascular system, reducing the risk of heart disease.

Risks and Considerations of Hormone Therapy

1. Breast Cancer Risk: Long-term use of combination hormone therapy (estrogen plus progestin) has been associated with a slightly increased risk of breast cancer.

2. Blood Clot Risk: Some types of hormone therapy, particularly oral forms, may increase the risk of blood clots, deep vein thrombosis, and stroke.

**3.	Hormone-Related	Cancers:** Long-term use of estrogen-alone therapy may increase the risk of endometrial (uterine) cancer.

4. Individualized Approach: The benefits and risks of hormone therapy vary based on factors such as age, health history, and the type of hormone therapy used.

Alternatives to Hormone Therapy

While hormone therapy is effective for symptom management, some women seek alternatives due to concerns about its potential risks. Several alternatives offer natural and non-hormonal approaches to managing menopausal symptoms:

1. Lifestyle Modifications

Healthy Diet: A diet rich in fruits, vegetables, whole grains, lean proteins, and healthy fats supports overall well-being and can alleviate certain symptoms.

Regular Exercise: Engaging in physical activity helps manage weight, improve mood, and reduce hot flashes.

Stress Reduction: Stress management techniques like meditation, yoga, and deep breathing can help alleviate mood swings and anxiety.

Adequate Sleep: Prioritizing quality sleep supports hormonal balance and overall health.

2. Herbal and Natural Supplements

Black Cohosh: This herbal supplement may alleviate hot flashes and mood swings in some women.

Soy and Flaxseed: These foods contain phytoestrogens that can provide mild relief for some menopausal symptoms.

Evening Primrose Oil: It is thought to help alleviate breast pain and irritability.

3. Cognitive Behavioral Therapy (CBT)

CBT can help manage mood disturbances, anxiety, and sleep disturbances often associated with menopause.

4. Vaginal Moisturizers and Lubricants

These products can alleviate vaginal dryness and discomfort without systemic hormonal effects.

5. Acupuncture

Some women find relief from menopausal symptoms, particularly hot flashes, through acupuncture sessions.

6. Bioidentical Hormones

Bioidentical hormones are synthesized to be chemically identical to the hormones naturally produced by the body.

They are often custom-compounded and may be perceived as more natural, but their safety and efficacy are still under debate.

Individualized Approach to Menopause Management

The journey through menopause is deeply personal, and there is no one-size-fits-all solution. What is effective for one woman might not be suitable for another. It's important to consult with a healthcare provider before making decisions about hormone therapy or alternative treatments. Factors to consider include:

1. Health History: Your medical history, including conditions such as breast cancer, cardiovascular disease, and blood clotting disorders.

2. Age and Menopausal Stage: The timing of menopause, as well as whether the uterus is intact, affects the suitability of hormone therapy.

3. Symptom Severity: The severity of symptoms and their impact on your daily life.

4. Personal Preferences: Your beliefs, values, and comfort level with different treatment options.

Informed Decision-Making

When considering hormone therapy or alternatives, it's important to engage in informed decision-making:

1. Consult a Healthcare Provider: Discuss your symptoms, concerns, and medical history with a healthcare provider. They can assist in identifying the most suitable strategy for your needs.

2. Weigh the Benefits and Risks: Understand the potential benefits and risks of each option. Consider how they align with your health goals and values.

3. Monitor and Reevaluate: If you choose a treatment option, regularly assess its effectiveness and make adjustments as needed.

4. Holistic Approach: Consider a holistic approach that combines lifestyle modifications, alternative therapies, and, if necessary, hormone therapy.

Hormone therapy and alternatives each have their benefits and considerations when it comes to managing menopause-related symptoms. The decision to pursue hormone therapy or explore alternative treatments is deeply personal and should be based on your individual health status, preferences, and needs. Consulting with a healthcare provider is essential to make informed choices that support your well-being during this transformative phase of life. Remember, whatever path you choose, it's a journey toward embracing menopause with empowerment, confidence, and vitality.

Chapter 6

Managing Bone and Joint Health

As women transition through menopause, a significant shift occurs in their hormonal balance, which can impact bone and joint health. The decline in estrogen levels during this phase can lead to a decrease in bone density and an increased risk of osteoporosis, while joint discomfort and stiffness may also become more prominent. Proactively managing bone and joint health becomes paramount during this time, as well as in the years that follow. By adopting a comprehensive approach that includes proper nutrition, exercise, lifestyle modifications, and medical guidance, women can maintain strong bones and healthy joints to support their overall well-being.

Understanding Bone Health During Menopause

Estrogen plays a critical role in maintaining bone density by supporting the activity of osteoblasts (cells that build bone) and inhibiting osteoclasts (cells that break down bone). When estrogen levels decrease, bone resorption may outpace bone formation, leading to a decline in bone mass and increasing the risk of fractures and osteoporosis.

1. Osteoporosis: Osteoporosis is a condition characterized by weakened and brittle bones, making them more susceptible to fractures. It often progresses silently until a fracture occurs, highlighting the importance of early prevention and management.

2. Bone Density Testing: Dual-energy X-ray absorptiometry (DXA) scans measure bone density and determine the risk of osteoporosis. Regular screenings can aid in early intervention.

Promoting Bone Health Through Nutrition

Nutrition plays a pivotal role in maintaining bone health. Essential nutrients support bone density and strength, contributing to overall skeletal integrity.

1. Calcium: Adequate calcium intake is crucial for bone health. Dairy items, enriched plant-based milk, green leafy vegetables, and nuts are exceptional sources.

2. Vitamin D: Vitamin D enhances calcium absorption. Sun exposure, fortified foods, fatty fish, and supplements contribute to vitamin D intake.

3. Magnesium: Magnesium supports bone mineralization. Whole grains, nuts, leafy greens, and seeds are magnesium-rich foods.

4. Vitamin K: Vitamin K aids in bone mineralization and supports bone health. Leafy greens, broccoli, and fermented foods are sources.

5. Protein: Protein supports bone health by providing essential amino acids. Incorporate fish, meats, lean, poultry, legumes, and beans.

6. Balanced Diet: A diet rich in fruits, vegetables, lean proteins, and whole grains provides comprehensive nutrition for bone health.

Exercising for Strong Bones and Joints

Exercise is a cornerstone of bone health, stimulating bone formation and enhancing bone density. Engaging in weight-bearing and resistance workouts is notably impactful.

1.   Weight-Bearing   Exercises: Activities that support body weight, such as walking, jogging, dancing, and stair climbing, promote bone health.

2. Strength Training: Resistance exercises, including lifting weights or using resistance bands, increase muscle strength and bone density.

3.   Balance   and   Coordination: Activities like yoga and tai chi improve balance and reduce the risk of falls and fractures.

4. Flexibility Exercises: Stretching and flexibility exercises maintain joint mobility and reduce the risk of joint stiffness.

Lifestyle Modifications for Bone and Joint Health

Lifestyle factors significantly impact bone and joint health. Simple changes can contribute to long-term well-being.

1. Quit Smoking: Smoking negatively affects bone health by reducing blood supply to bones and impeding healing.

2. Limit Alcohol: Excessive alcohol consumption can weaken bones and increase the risk of fractures.

3. Maintain a Healthy Weight: Maintaining a healthy weight reduces stress on joints and supports overall bone health.

4. Avoid Excessive Caffeine: High caffeine intake may interfere with calcium absorption.

5. Fall Prevention: Minimize the risk of falls by removing hazards at home, using handrails, and wearing proper footwear.

Seeking Medical Guidance

Regular healthcare check-ups are essential for bone and joint health. If needed, medical professionals can recommend appropriate interventions.

1. Medications: Some women may require medications to prevent or treat osteoporosis. Bisphosphonates, hormone therapy, and other medications are options.

2. Supplements: If dietary intake is insufficient, healthcare providers may recommend calcium or vitamin D supplements.

3. Physical Therapy: Physical therapists can provide exercises tailored to specific needs, alleviate joint pain, and improve mobility.

4. Pain Management: If joint discomfort persists, consult a healthcare provider for pain management strategies.

5. Hormone Therapy: Hormone therapy, under medical supervision, may be considered for bone health in specific cases.

Caring for Joints During Menopause

In addition to bone health, joint health is also a concern for women during menopause. Changes in hormonal balance and the natural aging process can contribute to joint discomfort, stiffness, and conditions such as osteoarthritis.

1. Regular Movement: Gentle, regular exercise helps maintain joint mobility and flexibility.

2. Weight Management: Maintaining a healthy weight reduces stress on joints, particularly weight-bearing ones like knees and hips.

3. Joint-Friendly Activities: Choose low-impact activities like swimming, cycling, and tai chi to minimize joint strain.

4. Warm-Up and Cool-Down: Prioritize warm-up exercises before engaging in physical activity and cool-down stretches afterward.

5. Proper Footwear: Wear supportive shoes that provide cushioning and reduce joint strain.

Managing bone and joint health is a proactive and ongoing journey that requires attention, care, and commitment. Women navigating menopause and the years beyond can take charge of their bone and joint health through a holistic approach that encompasses nutrition, exercise, lifestyle modifications, and medical guidance. By prioritizing these aspects of health, women can build a strong foundation for long-term well-being, supporting mobility, vitality, and an active lifestyle as they embrace the various chapters of life. Remember that investing in bone and joint health is an investment in your overall quality of life and independence.

Chapter 7

Heart and Sexual Health

As women transition through menopause, they experience significant hormonal changes that can impact various aspects of their health, including heart health and sexual well-being. The decline in estrogen levels during menopause can influence cardiovascular health and sexual function. Navigating these changes with a holistic approach that includes heart-healthy habits, open communication, and informed choices can empower women to maintain their overall well-being and quality of life during this transformative phase.

Understanding Heart Health During Menopause

Cardiovascular health becomes a paramount concern during menopause. Estrogen plays a protective role in the cardiovascular system by promoting healthy blood vessel function, reducing inflammation, and supporting healthy cholesterol levels. As estrogen levels decline, the risk of heart disease increases.

1. Heart Disease: The risk of heart disease rises post-menopause, with factors such as high blood pressure, high cholesterol, and excess weight contributing to this risk.

2. Hypertension: Blood pressure tends to rise during menopause, increasing the risk of hypertension.

3. Cholesterol Levels: LDL cholesterol (often referred to as "bad" cholesterol) may increase, while HDL cholesterol (often referred to as "good" cholesterol) may decrease.

4. **Inflammation:** Chronic inflammation is associated with heart disease, and hormonal changes during menopause can contribute to increased inflammation.

Promoting Heart Health Through Lifestyle

Adopting heart-healthy lifestyle habits can have a significant impact on cardiovascular well-being during and after menopause.

1. Balanced Diet: Emphasize a diet rich in fruits, vegetables, whole grains, lean proteins, and healthy fats.

Reduce the intake of saturated and trans fats, sodium, and added sugars.

2. Consistent Physical Activity: Participate in routine bodily movements, encompassing aerobic routines, muscle-strengthening exercises, and flexibility training.

3. Weight Management: Maintaining a healthy weight reduces the risk of heart disease and supports overall well-being.

4. Blood Pressure Control: Monitor blood pressure regularly and work with a healthcare provider to manage hypertension.

5. Cholesterol Management: If cholesterol levels are high, work with a healthcare provider to develop a plan for managing cholesterol through diet, exercise, and, if necessary, medication.

6. Stress Reduction: Chronic stress contributes to heart disease risk. Utilize stress-relieving methods such as meditation, deep breathing, and mindfulness practices.

7. Adequate Sleep: Prioritize quality sleep, as sleep plays a role in heart health and overall well-being.

8. Avoid Smoking and Limit Alcohol: Quit smoking and limit alcohol consumption to promote heart health.

Sexual Health and Intimacy

Maintaining sexual well-being is a crucial component of overall health and one's quality of life. During menopause, hormonal changes can influence sexual desire, arousal, lubrication, and satisfaction.

1. Vaginal Changes: Declining estrogen levels can lead to vaginal dryness and thinning of vaginal tissues, causing discomfort during intercourse.

2. Libido: Changes in hormone levels can impact sexual desire or libido.

3. Emotional Factors: Mood changes, stress, and body image concerns can also affect sexual well-being.

Communication and Open Dialogue

Open communication with a partner and healthcare provider is key to addressing sexual health concerns during menopause.

1. Partner Communication: Discuss your feelings, concerns, and desires with your partner to maintain intimacy and connection.

2. Healthcare Provider: If experiencing discomfort or changes in sexual health, discuss these concerns with a healthcare provider. Solutions may include vaginal moisturizers, lubricants, or hormonal therapies.

3. Mental and Emotional Health: Address mood changes or anxiety that may affect sexual well-being. Obtaining therapy or counseling can offer assistance and guidance.

Hormone Therapy and Sexual Health

For some women, hormone therapy may positively impact sexual health by alleviating symptoms such as vaginal dryness and low libido. Hormone therapy is a personal decision and should be discussed with a healthcare provider.

1. Local Hormone Therapy: Estrogen-based vaginal creams, rings, or tablets can help relieve vaginal dryness and discomfort.

2. Systemic Hormone Therapy: Hormone therapy, such as estrogen and/or progesterone, can address overall menopausal symptoms, potentially improving sexual well-being.

Navigating heart health and sexual well-being during menopause requires a comprehensive and holistic approach. By prioritizing heart-healthy habits, managing cardiovascular risk factors, and fostering open communication about sexual health, women can empower themselves to embrace this transformative phase with vitality and confidence. It's essential to remember that individual experiences vary, and what works for one woman may differ for another.

Chapter 8

Self-Care and Emotional Well-being

Menopause is a transformative journey that encompasses both physical changes and emotional shifts. As women navigate this phase, prioritizing self-care and emotional well-being becomes essential for maintaining overall health and quality of life. The hormonal fluctuations and life adjustments that accompany menopause can impact mental and emotional health. By embracing self-care practices and fostering emotional resilience, women can navigate this journey with grace, empowerment, and a renewed sense of self.

Emotional Wellbeing During Menopause

The hormonal changes that occur during menopause can influence mood, emotions, and overall mental health. Estrogen plays a role in neurotransmitter regulation, and its decline can contribute to mood swings, irritability, and anxiety.

1. Mood Swings: Fluctuations in hormone levels can lead to sudden shifts in mood and emotional state.

2. Anxiety and Depression: Some women experience increased anxiety or depressive symptoms during menopause, which can be exacerbated by hormonal changes and life transitions.

3. Sleep Disturbances: Sleep disruptions are common during menopause and can contribute to emotional and mood changes.

4. Self-Esteem and Body Image:

Physical changes may impact self-esteem and body image, affecting emotional well-being.

Prioritizing Self-Care

Self-care involves intentional actions that promote physical, mental, and emotional health. Prioritizing self-care is vital for managing the emotional challenges that may arise during menopause.

1. Physical Self-Care

Healthy Diet: Provide your body with nourishing foods that contribute to your overall well-being and health.

Regular Exercise: Engage in regular physical activity to boost mood, reduce stress, and support physical health.

Adequate Sleep: Prioritize quality sleep to support mood regulation and emotional resilience.

Hydration: Stay hydrated to support cognitive function and overall health.

2. Mental and Emotional Self-Care

Mindfulness and Meditation: Engage in mindfulness techniques to remain in the present moment and alleviate stress, while meditation promotes emotional equilibrium.

Journaling: Writing down your thoughts and feelings can provide clarity, release emotions, and promote self-awareness.

Therapy or Counseling: Seek professional support if emotional challenges become overwhelming. Therapy offers tools to cope with stress, anxiety, and mood fluctuations.

Positive Affirmations: Use positive affirmations to cultivate self-compassion and boost self-esteem.

Limit Screen Time: Reduce exposure to negative or stressful content online to protect your emotional well-being.

3. Social Self-Care

Social Connections: Maintain relationships with friends and loved ones for emotional support and connection.

Setting Boundaries: Set boundaries to protect your emotional energy and prevent burnout.

Engage in Activities You Enjoy: Participate in hobbies and activities that bring you joy and provide a sense of accomplishment.

4. Creative Self-Care

Art and Creative Expression: Engage in artistic activities that allow you to express emotions and enhance your sense of self.

Music and Dance: Music and dance can be uplifting and therapeutic, improving mood and emotional well-being.

Cultivating Emotional Resilience

Emotional resilience involves the ability to adapt to challenges, cope with stress, and bounce back from adversity. Building emotional resilience is essential for navigating the emotional changes of menopause.

1. **Practice Mindfulness:** Mindfulness techniques, such as deep breathing and grounding exercises, can help you stay present and manage stress.

2. Embrace Change: Accept that menopause is a natural life transition. Embracing change can reduce the stress associated with resisting the inevitable.

3. Seek Support: Connect with friends, family, or support groups to share experiences and receive emotional support.

4. Challenge Negative Thoughts: Practice cognitive reframing to challenge negative thought patterns and cultivate a positive mindset.

5. Self-Compassion: Treat yourself with kindness and understanding, especially during times of emotional struggle.

6. Cultivate Gratitude: Focusing on gratitude can shift your perspective and improve emotional well-being.

<u>Navigating Emotional Challenges</u>

Emotional challenges are a natural part of the menopause journey. It's crucial to acknowledge when the assistance of a professional is required.

1. Recognize When to Seek Help: If feelings of sadness, anxiety, or mood changes become overwhelming, seek the guidance of a mental health professional.

2. Therapy Options: Cognitive-behavioral therapy (CBT), talk therapy, and other therapeutic approaches can provide tools to manage emotional challenges.

3. Medication: In some cases, medication may be recommended to manage severe emotional symptoms. Consult a healthcare provider for guidance.

Strengthening Emotional Bonds in Relationships

Menopause can impact relationships due to mood swings, emotional changes, and physical symptoms.

Open communication and mutual support are crucial.

1. Communication: Openly discuss emotional changes and challenges with loved ones to foster understanding and empathy.

2. Mutual Support: Encourage open dialogue about emotional well-being and provide mutual support during challenging times.

3. Empathy: Practice empathy and active listening to create a supportive and safe environment for emotional expression.

4. Couples Counseling: Consider couples counseling to address emotional challenges and strengthen your relationship.

Embracing self-care and fostering emotional well-being are integral components of navigating the menopause journey with resilience and empowerment. By prioritizing physical health, engaging in mindfulness practices, seeking professional support when needed, and cultivating emotional resilience, women can navigate the emotional changes of menopause and emerge stronger, more self-aware, and better equipped to face life's challenges.

Remember that self-care is not selfish; it's a necessary investment in your mental, emotional, and overall well-being as you embrace the various phases of this transformative journey.

Chapter 9

Thriving Beyond Menopause

Menopause marks a significant transition in a woman's life, signifying the end of reproductive years and the beginning of a new chapter. While it brings physical and hormonal changes, menopause also offers an opportunity for personal growth, self-discovery, and renewed vitality. Thriving beyond menopause involves embracing this phase with a positive mindset, maintaining health and well-being, nurturing personal passions, and fostering meaningful connections. By approaching menopause as a gateway to new possibilities rather than a limitation, women can create a vibrant and fulfilling life that extends well beyond this transformative journey.

1. Embracing Change and Transformation

Menopause is a natural and unavoidable aspect of a woman's life journey. Embracing this transition with acceptance and a positive mindset sets the stage for thriving beyond menopause. Acknowledge that change is a constant in life, and menopause is a new phase filled with potential. Instead of focusing on what is ending, shift your perspective to what is beginning.

2. Prioritizing Physical Health

Maintaining physical health is key to thriving beyond menopause. A healthy body supports overall well-being and allows you to fully engage in life's opportunities.

Balanced Diet: Nourish your body with a diet rich in fruits, vegetables, lean proteins, whole grains, and healthy fats. Adequate nutrition fuels your energy and vitality.

Regular Exercise: Engage in regular physical activity that suits your preferences, whether it's walking, yoga, swimming, or dancing. Exercise enhances mood, boosts energy, and supports overall health.

Bone and Joint Health: Focus on bone health to prevent osteoporosis by incorporating weight-bearing exercises and adequate calcium and vitamin D intake.

Heart Health: Prioritize heart health through healthy lifestyle choices to reduce the risk of cardiovascular disease.

Adequate Sleep: Prioritize restful sleep to support cognitive function, mood, and overall health.

3. Nurturing Emotional Wellbeing

Cultivating emotional resilience and self-care practices contribute to a positive and fulfilling post-menopausal life.

Mindfulness: Practice mindfulness and meditation to stay present, manage stress, and enhance emotional balance.

Self-Compassion: Treat yourself with kindness and self-compassion. Embrace imperfections and celebrate your achievements.

Seek Support: If emotional challenges arise, seek support from friends, family, or a mental health professional.

Engage in Creative Activities: Creative expression through art, writing, music, or other hobbies can provide a therapeutic outlet for emotions.

4. Pursuing Passions and Interests

Thriving beyond menopause involves pursuing personal passions and interests that bring joy and fulfillment.

Lifelong Learning: Explore new interests, take up a hobby, or enroll in classes that stimulate your mind and keep you engaged.

Professional Goals: Consider career shifts or new challenges, embracing the wisdom and experience you've gained.

Travel and Exploration: Embark on adventures and travel to places you've always wanted to visit. Exploring new environments can invigorate the spirit.

5. Fostering Relationships and Connections

Nurturing meaningful relationships contributes to a fulfilling post-menopausal life.

Maintain Friendships: Cultivate existing friendships and create opportunities to meet new people who share your interests.

Family Bonds: Strengthen relationships with family members and enjoy the rewarding role of being a parent or grandparent.

Romantic Relationships: If you're in a romantic relationship, continue to nurture emotional and physical intimacy.

6. Mindset Shift: From Menopause to Meno-empowerment

Reframe how you view menopause. Instead of considering it as a decline, view it as an opportunity for empowerment and growth.

Wisdom: Menopause brings wisdom and experience gained over the years.

Embrace this wisdom and share it with others.

Freedom: Embrace the freedom that comes with not having to worry about reproductive concerns. Redirect this energy into other areas of your life.

Self-Discovery: Menopause offers an opportunity for self-discovery and introspection. Reflect on your values, goals, and aspirations.

Resilience: The challenges you've faced and overcome throughout life have cultivated resilience. Apply this resilience to thrive beyond menopause.

Thriving beyond menopause is a mindset, a conscious decision to embrace this phase with positivity, resilience, and a commitment to self-care. By prioritizing physical health, nurturing emotional well-being, pursuing passions, fostering connections, and shifting your mindset, you can create a vibrant and fulfilling life that extends well beyond menopause. Remember that life's journey is filled with various chapters, and menopause is just one of them. Embrace this chapter with enthusiasm, knowing that it's a stepping stone to a future filled with possibilities, growth, and continued joy. As you navigate the years beyond menopause, you have the power to shape your narrative and create a life that truly reflects your inner strength and vitality.

www.ingramcontent.com/pod-product-compliance
Lightning Source LLC
Chambersburg PA
CBHW071605270726
48661CB00018B/1249